UNDERSTANDING AUTISM IN KIDS

The ultimate guide to understanding autism in toddlers

Robert T. Moon

Table of content

Chapter 1: What Is Autism?

There is no one type of autism, but many.

A wide variety of diseases collectively known as autism, or autistic spectrum disorder (ASD), are characterized by difficulties with social skills, repetitive activities, speech, and nonverbal communication. The Centers for Disease Control estimate that 1 in 44 American children currently suffer from autism.

We are aware that there are several subtypes of autism, the majority of which are driven by a confluence of hereditary and environmental variables. Since autism is a spectrum condition, each autistic individual has a unique set of abilities and difficulties. People with autism can learn, reason, and solve problems in a variety of ways, from highly proficient to severely impaired. While some persons with ASD could need a lot of everyday assistance, others might just need a little help and in some circumstances might even live independently.

Autism may be caused by a variety of circumstances, and it frequently coexists with sensory sensitivities, physical conditions including gastrointestinal (GI) diseases, seizures, or sleep disorders, as well as psychological difficulties like anxiety, depression, and attention deficits.

Autism symptoms often manifest around the age of 2 or 3. Some related developmental impairments may manifest much sooner, and they are frequently detectable as early as 18 months. According to research, early intervention helps autistic persons achieve their goals later in life.

* The American Psychiatric Association combined four separate diagnoses of autism into one overarching diagnosis of autism spectrum disorder in 2013. (ASD). They included Asperger syndrome, pervasive

developmental disorder-not otherwise defined (PDD-NOS), childhood disintegrative disorder, and autistic disorder.

What Are the Three Levels of Autism?

The Diagnostic and Statistical Manual of Mental Disorders, Fifth Edition, defines the different levels of autism spectrum disorder (ASD) (DSM-5). Three distinct levels are provided by the 5th edition criteria for diagnosing autism based on the patient's support needs. These stages of autism enable doctors to establish more precise diagnoses, enabling more efficient treatment programs and assisting caregivers in better comprehending the symptoms and requirements of individuals.

ASD Level 1: Requiring Support

The mildest or "highest functioning" type of autism, known as Level 1, affects those who would have previously received an Asperger's syndrome diagnosis. People with

ASD level 1 may struggle to build and sustain personal relationships as well as struggle to recognize social cues. A child with level 1 autism may comprehend and talk in entire phrases, but they may find it challenging to converse back and forth.

Some inflexibility of behavior, such as trouble transitioning between tasks, remaining organized, and planning, is experienced by children with ASD level 1 disorders.

ASD Level 2: Requiring Substantial Support

Children with level 2 ASDs display social communication and repetitive behaviors more overtly than children with level 1 autism. Children at this level struggle with verbal and nonverbal communication, and they also respond less or strangely to social cues.

Additionally, the inflexibility of behavior is more obvious than it is in ASD level 1.

Repeated behaviors are more noticeable and can be seen by casual observers. Similarly, youngsters with level 2 autism may struggle to adjust to changes in routine, which may result in challenging behavior.

ASD Level 3: Requiring Very Substantial Support

Significant difficulties in social contact and incredibly rigid conduct are characteristics of ASD level 3. Children with level 3 autism will either be nonverbal or utilize a limited number of understandable words. Both initiating social interactions and responding to others are exceedingly rare. At this stage, social interactions with others could be aberrant and limited to urgent requirements.

People with level 3 autism have considerable behavioral rigidity and have a very difficult time adapting to changes in routine. At this stage, the person's capacity to function is hampered by restricted or repeated habits.

Switching your attention from one task to another may be quite challenging and distressing.

Five subcategories of autism were defined in the previous diagnostic manual (DSM-IV), from Asperger's syndrome (mild, or high-functioning autism) to autistic disorder (severe autism), which are now regarded as out-of-date diagnoses. Rett syndrome and childhood disintegrative disorder (CDD), two uncommon disorders that are no longer regarded as being on the autism spectrum, were also included.

Myths and misconceptions

People with autism spectrum disorders may find it challenging to have their illness recognized and to get the support they require due to a lack of understanding.

Some autistic people may experience loneliness and isolation as a result of misconceptions. In extreme circumstances, it may also result in bullying and abuse.

There are many myths and misunderstandings surrounding autism spectrum disorder.
Autism is an illness that has historically been greatly misunderstood, from the idea of "refrigerator mothers" to the notion that every person with autism is like "Rain Man."

Many myths and misunderstandings still exist today.
The top five myths, in my opinion, are listed below, along with an explanation of the actual reality!

Myth: Vaccinations cause autism

There is just no scientific evidence to support this despite the fact that numerous large-scale, gold-standard scientific investigations have been conducted.
If it were so easy, we would already be aware. The complex condition of autism

appears to be brought on by a wide range of genetic and environmental factors. The promise of an immediate solution, an easy way to solve the problem, or even a speedy cure has lured many parents.

Life is unfortunately not simple, but rest assured that great efforts are being done to elucidate the genes and other contributing variables in order to better understand autism and effectively treat its symptoms.

Myth: Autistic children don't want to make friends.

Most of the time, simply untrue. Some young individuals and adults opt to keep a significant distance from other people and are very distant. However, the majority of children and adults with autism do like interacting with others.

Our kids' social skills are lacking, and as a result, they frequently make mistakes. Being social is like learning a really difficult dance, and it frequently calls for quick thinking. It can seem impossible. Our kids can learn the dance, though, if we slow it down and describe the moves.

People on the spectrum may experience extreme anxiety when engaging in social situations, especially if they have previously failed. However, the desire to connect is frequently present, and it is up to family, school, and therapists to support our loved ones in successfully interacting with others.

Myth: Autistic children are unable to learn.

They can, without a doubt, if the rest of us learn how to teach them effectively. Most kids will get better with treatment, but it has to be good therapy that is made just for that kid.

For some people, learning is challenging, and they will make very slow progress.

Still, if family and teachers are persistent and employ a successful teaching strategy, things can change and lives can get better slowly but surely.

Myth: Poor parenting causes autism

I'm sorry, but it's not. Autism cannot be caused by bad parenting, yet it cannot be helped for any child.

Because our children are not responding to us as a regularly developing youngster would, many parents feel that we are not doing a good job of being parents. If I have multiple children and just one of them has autism, this is so obvious.

I can, however, raise all of our children to be good parents. And the more I comprehend our kids, the more room they have to grow.

Myth: People with autism are savants, like Rain Man.

Not everyone is able to name everyone in the phone book or tell someone they meet on their birthday. There are some people who can perform incredible memory feats, but this is uncommon.

Many autistic children do have some strengths in common, such as the ability to learn visually or to retain visual information well. Children can use these advantages to assist them get around in the world.

Contrary to pseudoscience
It can be quite difficult to accept the news that your child has autism when it is first discovered. The future of your child may appear uncertain and the road ahead looks overwhelming.

Some parents may then turn to pseudoscientific therapies in an effort to find a "fast fix" or a cure for their autistic child (learn more about autism cures).

What then is pseudoscience? It is described by Wikipedia as "anything that claims to be science but is not." In other words, it is "false science."

When a theory or notion is taken and a rigorous experiment is designed to evaluate if it is true (or not), that is good science.

A controlled clinical trial is one method I can do this. In a controlled trial, two closely matched groups—say, let's two groups of preschoolers with autism—are compared with the intervention being tested (for instance, a novel kind of therapy) and another treatment (or no treatment).

Exclusively the therapy differs between the two groups in a well-designed trial, so if positive improvements are only observed in that group, I may be relatively confident that I am observing an effect from that treatment.

To ensure the same outcomes are discovered, the trial should ideally be repeated at least once (preferably by a separate team of researchers). Treatments that go through this kind of extensive testing are referred to as "evidence-based."

Pseudoscientists tend to employ a lot of scientific terminology, and their views might first be very persuasive. They are less interested in proving that their "therapy" is effective or not. They can even claim that controlled trials are not required.

The following are further indicators of pseudoscience. Watch out for anyone promoting:

Everything they say will cure autism: Autism currently has no known cure. In fact, some people think I shouldn't be looking for one, and the idea offends a lot of people.
It is incomprehensible that top authorities on autism be in the dark about the existence of a treatment. If there is a significant development in the treatment of autism, it

will be tremendous international news and everyone will be aware of it!

Therapies built on overly simple notions: The complex illness of autism has a strong genetic component and alters how the brain is wired. It's highly improbable that only one reason will ever be identified.
There is insufficient evidence to support the claims that people with autism may be cured with elimination diets alone or that their aberrant biochemistry necessitates the use of pricey supplements.

They offer treatments that they say work well for utterly unrelated illnesses: What are the connections between cancer and autism? Nearly nothing. However, certain medical procedures are marketed as cures for both ailments.
Treatments whose efficacy is solely attested to by personal experiences or testimonies: Truthfully determining whether a treatment

is effective or not requires well planned trials.

any medical procedure that states it has no negative effects. Nothing is without side effects, and certain therapies can even be time-wasting or even dangerous at their worst.

conspiracy ideas Take caution if someone suggests a medical procedure that "doctors don't want to inform you about."

Like everyone else, doctors desire the best results for autistic individuals. In reality, a lot of doctors are also parents. There is no logical explanation for why they would withhold from you effective therapies.

I strongly advise you to consult a reputable healthcare provider before beginning any treatment that raises one or more of these warning signs.

Keep in mind the sage advice:

"If it sounds too good to be true, it probably is"

While only a small percentage of these treatments will actually hurt your child, they can definitely harm your bank account. More significantly, embracing pseudoscience can divert you from seeking out treatments for your child that are supported by evidence.

ASD Complications

You might have sensory issues, seizures, mental health issues, or other issues if you have ASD.

Sensory issues
You might be extremely sensitive to sensory input if you have ASD. Even ordinary things like loud noises or bright lights might make you feel quite uncomfortable emotionally. As an alternative, some sensations, such

intense heat, cold, or discomfort, may have no effect on you at all.

Seizures
ASD sufferers frequently experience seizures. They frequently start when you're young or in your teen years.

Difficulties with mental health
The risk of melancholy, anxiety, impulsive behavior, and mood swings increases if you have ASD.

Mental illness
There is some degree of mental impairment in many ASD sufferers. The risk of ASD in children with fragile X syndrome is higher. A X chromosomal segment has an abnormality that results in this condition. It frequently leads to mental disability, especially in boys.

Tumors

A uncommon condition called tuberous sclerosis makes benign tumors grow in your organs, including your brain. Uncertain is the relationship between ASD and tuberous sclerosis. However, compared to children without the illness, children with tuberous sclerosis had much greater rates of ASD, according to the Centers for Disease Control and Prevention (Trusted Source).

Other difficulties
Aggression, strange sleeping, eating, and digestive disorders are some other symptoms that can come along with ASD.

Chapter 2: Autism First Signs: A Checklist for Babies and Toddlers

Autism Awareness Month is in April. According to the advocacy organization Autism Speaks, the illness, which affects 1 in 68 children, is the most rapidly expanding significant developmental impairment in the United States.

Although there is no known cure for autism spectrum disorders (ASD), early identification and treatment can significantly enhance the lives of afflicted children and their families. ASD cannot be detected with a medical test. Instead, professionals evaluate a child's evolving social and behavioral abilities, frequently starting as early as 12 months.

Instead of using any biological testing, a diagnosis of autism is established based on a collection of criteria. This is one of the factors contributing to the difficulty in diagnosing a kid with autism until they are between 18 and 22 months old (although some of the signs of autism may be noticed before the age of 1).

Milestones and development

The rate at which children acquire new behaviors and abilities as they mature naturally varies from kid to child. However, there are several developmental milestones that infants and young children may be anticipated to accomplish in an usual or average amount of time.

Although this won't always be the case, since there are many factors that can affect a newborn's development, if a baby develops at a noticeably different rate or shows major variances in their style of growing when compared to others their age, they may be on the autism spectrum.

This list of symptoms and traits may be useful for parents or caregivers of a kid whose rate of development differs from that of their classmates and who is suspected to have autism.

The ASDetect app also offers films that highlight some of the traits of autism in infants and toddlers, making it an additional helpful resource for parents and caregivers.

The checklists and app are only suggestions, it is crucial to keep in mind, and medical experts are educated to be able to spot symptoms of developmental disparities in infants. Any worries you may have should be raised with a professional, since only a trained diagnostician is able to make an autism diagnosis.

Signs and characteristics of autism in babies checklist

These are some common characteristics of autism that may be observed in babies and young children, although it is unlikely that a child will show signs of all of them. Some signs may change over time, or become more obvious as a child gets older.

Early signs of autism in babies (6 months to one year) may include:

- Reacting in an unexpected way to new faces
- Rarely smiling in social situations
- Making little or no eye contact
- Difficulty in following objects with their eyes
- Hearing their name does not produce a response
- Having limited or no reaction to loud sounds, or not turning their head to locate sounds
- Overreacting to some sounds

- Displaying a lack of interest in interactive games, like peek-a-boo
- Chattering, or imitating sounds and words is limited
- Gestures like pointing at an object they want or waving back at others are limited
- Tendency not to imitate the actions of other people
- Dislike of being touched or cuddled, or not reaching out when about to be picked up, or
- Displaying unusual or repetitive body movements.
- Early signs of autism in toddlers up to 24 months may include:
- Limited or no speech
- Only walking on their toes
- Difficulty in following simple verbal instructions
- Gestures and imitating others' actions are limited
- Showing an intense interest in certain objects, at the exclusion of all else

- Showing an intense interest in unusual or unexpected objects or materials
- Unwillingness to share objects or activities they are interested in, or to engage the attention of others, or
- Engaging in repetitive actions and activities, such as putting objects into lines or groups, etc.

Early signs of autism in young children up to 36 months may include:

- Limited speech
- Difficulties in being able to follow simple verbal instructions
- Showing little interest in imaginative play, such as pretend games
- Showing little interest in other children
- Wanting routines to be followed and being upset by change

- Extreme sensitivity to sight, sound, smell, taste and some other sensory experiences
- Displaying limited or no sensitivity to some sensory experiences such as heat, cold, touch, hunger, thirst or pain, or
- Becoming fixated on playing with particular toys, activities or actions.

Should I get an autism assessment for my baby?

It is important to remember that these are signs and characteristics that babies and toddlers with autism may display, but they are by no means definitive, and their presence or absence should not be taken by parents or carers as conclusive evidence of autism or otherwise.

Instead, if your baby or toddler displays some of the characteristics of autism outlined above, or is developing at a different rate to other children of their age, it is important that you get the advice of a medical professional, such as your GP, a nurse or a health worker.

Chapter 3: Do's & Don'ts

How To handle An Autistic Child

Parents, teachers, and guardians who are caring for or helping children with autism may become frustrated by having to deal with their behavior.

Such actions may occur suddenly or persist for a long time. Anyone may find it challenging to maintain control and create humiliation, especially while in public.

However, some autistic children like conversing with their relatives, acquaintances, or other individuals they meet outdoors.

When someone discusses or displays photos of something they are enthusiastic about, this is more likely to happen.

It can sometimes happen that they talk for too long, irritating the people around them, including the parents.

The information provided below explains how people, and parents in particular, may deal with the undesired behaviors associated with children who have autism more effectively.

Aggression, self-harm, irritating behaviors like tantrums, or even talkativeness are examples of this. Since dealing with children with ASD can be difficult, preparation is essential.

But having a plan of action and exercises to complete can help you feel less frustrated.

So continue reading to discover the most effective methods for soothing down and correcting an autistic youngster.

1 Calming Them Down

Children with autism are more prone to tantrums. Nevertheless, parents can only manage them for so long before they start to feel overburdened.

This is a difficulty for parents, teachers, and others who don't have regular contact with the youngster. Everyone has a certain amount of tolerance, but how aggressive and unpleasant conduct is handled may greatly ease coping with it.

Tantrums in autistic children could eventually start to happen often and continue no matter where they are.

For the youngsters as well as the parents, teachers, or anybody else there at the time, it can be a frightening event.

The surroundings of an autistic kid, including their siblings, should be safe, and parents should make it a priority.

Struggling with aggressiveness can be difficult for parents, but it helps to understand it better when you try to figure out what triggers strong emotions in children with ASD. Management is much made easier if these are identified.

Anyone can be the subject of such hostile action, although peers are frequently targeted.

They are the most inclined to confront repetitious behaviors or alter their routine.

Since they frequently want to change their activities, caregivers of the kid are also frequently aggressive. Therapists may have this issue with children who have significant symptoms.

A large portion of the aggression is caused by autistic children acting out their urges.

They are not anticipated before they take place. Their responses are spontaneous, spur-of-the-moment events that they have no intention in initiating.

Some autistic youngsters do, however, act aggressively to acquire what they want. Parents or other caregivers may give in to a child's conduct because they find it soothing or distracting after an outburst.

Long-term harm might result from this because they can become more aggressive if the activity or behavior is abruptly stopped. A typical reaction is to bang one's head.

When parents are angry, they should maintain their composure.
When children see their parents behaving adversely, it may be assumed that what they

are doing is normal since it may seem to be the same as how they are acting.

The most crucial step in helping an autistic kid comprehend why their behaviors are inappropriate may be teaching them how to control their own behavior in stressful situations.

Here are some other strategies parents may use to handle tantrums:

Have a well-executed plan in place

For children who become overwhelmed easily, a strategy should be set up so they will know what to do when the anxiety strikes.Some of them may even be made fun or simple to do. For instance, if a youngster notices that their anxiety is increasing, they can tell their parents what is happening and count up or down to a certain amount. Children who aren't yet developed enough to count higher should start with counting to 10, which can simultaneously help them learn about numbers and reduce tension.

Also known as toys that engage the child's senses. They are often simple to locate in most stores that offer kids' toys.This works well with balls or other fluffy, squishy, and squeeze-able objects. Clay is also suggested, albeit not as much for those with carpeted floors. They can also use fidget spinners to deal with their nervousness. Purchase a trampoline, either indoors or out. Trampolines are fantastic for connecting and helping them relieve tension when they are experiencing overwhelming emotions. They are useful for self-regulation. They can assist with self-regulation and sensory intake. Outdoor trampolines are typically available at big box shops or online, whereas indoor trampolines are typically found in toy stores.

Have them put on a blanket or a vest;

Any vest will not do. Use one that is comfortable to wear and has a moderate amount of weight. Children with autism may feel more at ease when they are heavy, which can help them deal with situations where they are most likely to experience sensory overload, such as during school hours. As long as it's not too hot outside, other gathering spots are appropriate for a weighted blanket or clothing items.

Buy chewable pencil and pen tips

Giving an autistic youngster something to chew on may be all that's required to help them feel at ease and act normally. Parents should only do this with children who have the self-control to refrain from chewing on all writing implements as a result of being given chewable substitutes.

Investigate more drug options

This can be interpreted as giving a kid medicine that hasn't been prescribed to them by a physician or other healthcare provider, or that the FDA hasn't approved. But when kids demonstrate an interest in such topics, practices like meditation can be effective. If they see their loved ones using meditation techniques, kids may become more receptive to them. They can learn how to be mindful and use different breathing techniques to promote relaxation through meditation, which is very helpful. They can incorporate meditation practice into a game to help them cope with stress or agitation.

Think about getting a pet

It is acceptable to get a pet, but parents must teach their kids how to interact with the animal and prevent any harm.The ability of dogs and cats to calm autistic children is one of the reasons some parents choose to supplement their child's regular ABA sessions with animal therapy.

2 Getting Them To Listen

It takes time to teach a youngster with autism how to listen more effectively. There are no hard and fast rules in this, however some families have found success by using the following guidance:

1. Becoming more patient

Children with ASD typically progress through learning at a different rate than other kids their age. This also entails how they process fresh information as it is received.

Parents should take every precaution to make sure that their children aren't learning new things too rapidly by pushing them to do so.

Stopping can assist them have enough time to hear, process, and respond to what is being said.

This issue may also be seen in kids without any diseases. It affects everyone, not just those with ASD.

Their mental health and confidence in learning and trying out new things to prevent meltdowns can both benefit from knowing that they have patient parents, instructors, and friends who are there to help.

2. Maintain an optimistic outlook
Children with autism respond well when they receive a lot of encouragement from the individuals they engage with.

Even when children show signs of worry and tension, parents should maintain a kind tone in their presence.

3. Interact with them physically to communicate.
Short attention spans are a common sign of ASD. They may find it challenging to communicate since they frequently become distracted.

However, when an effort is made to speak with a kid while they are engaged in play, some youngsters can improve their comprehension.

In this case, physical exercise can be performed both indoors and outside. They ought to be allowed to play inside in an area where they may roam around freely without hurting anything or themselves.

4. Demonstrate love
Affection is another sort of positive reinforcement, particularly when it comes from a child's parent, pet, friends, or other family members.

A hug or pat on the back should be given to them anytime they behave well at school, in public, or at home as they may need affection more than the ordinary youngster.

Furthermore, if they are in a mood where affection is ineffective, it is OK to give them some of their own space.

5. Express your interest in them to them.
Children with autism frequently struggle to communicate with others.

Parents should continually convey to their children that they are in their thoughts and are significant, either via verbal or nonverbal cues, to help them understand that they are not alone in their feelings.

6. Learn with them.
Even by applying the rules governing how it is handled to aid in coping with challenges on their own, parents may learn a lot about children with autism.

Their unique requirements can spark discussion and teach individuals new ways to engage with others and solve issues by remaining composed and open to dialogue.

7. Participating in or planning a support group
Children with autism are highly advised to join support groups. It might make parents feel less alone and enable them to network with others in their community to learn more about reputable rehabilitation facilities.

How to discipline children with autism

Tell them that there are rewards and penalties for the things they do.

One of the principles of ABA treatment is this, thus a therapist from a facility may assist parents in better understanding disciplinary procedures and learning when to provide positive reinforcement.

The road that provides children with the positive reinforcement they love so much from behaving nicely should be guided.

When engaging in undesirable behavior, students should be aware of the repercussions, which may include receiving less rewards.

How To Avoid Losing Patience With An Autistic Child

If parents are frustrated or irritated with their autistic child's conduct, they should seek therapy for themselves.

But most importantly, they need to keep a cheerful outlook no matter what.
By keeping in mind the benefit of excellent behavior, they may encourage their child.

When someone behaves nicely, they should receive praise from everyone they know.

They can now distinguish between suitable and inappropriate behavior thanks to this.

Parental patience is maintained via communication.

If this doesn't work, parents should try to identify additional concerns, such as health-related issues or stressful events at work, that may be making them feel impatient or irritated with their child.

What Not To Do With An Autistic Child

What not to do while dealing with kids that have autism is as follows:

Feeding into their behavior - Children with autism spectrum disorders may interact with parents or caregivers by making obnoxious noises or moving in ways they believe would attract their attention.
If kids notice that it gets them what they want, it could turn into bad behavior. Since

there wouldn't be a good response or reaction to the conduct, the youngster is on the road to learning why it shouldn't be done by choosing to ignore it.

Considering they are unable to converse - All children with ASD can communicate, however some may find it easier to do so in writing or by other non-verbal ways.

Don't push them to create eye contact; autistic children often have trouble doing so. Although it is a lengthy procedure that shouldn't be imposed, they may be trained to gaze towards the forehead.

Chapter 4: Practical Tips to Raising A Child With Autism

Here are a few strategies that are helping families to cope:

1. Reframe acting-out behaviors.
Many children with ASD, suffer from sensory integration challenges and become unglued within minutes of entering buildings. Every child has a different threshold for sensory overload, and each child develops new skills at different ages. If entering highly occupied buildings like malls triggers your child and you notice they aren't yet ready for that experience. Visiting smaller retail stores with less sensory stimuli can prove to be a much more successful endeavor.

2. Use positive discipline.
For many children, positive feedback and encouragement can be a motivating and very effective form of discipline. The same is

true for children on the spectrum. All too often, parents fall into the trap of monitoring and correcting behaviors without always acknowledging when their child is displaying positive actions. Well-placed compliments and expressions of love went a long way in building their self-confidence and promoting constructive behaviors.

3. Celebrate quirks and talents.
Strengths typically represent your ASD child's highest-functioning area. We now have a greater awareness of many famous and accomplished individuals in the arts and entertainment world who have ASD. Several of them are award-winning musicians and directors! Recognizing your child's talents and reinforcing them is key. Rather than just attending to areas of deficit, focus on your child's strengths. One helpful tip is to redirect repetitive play and interests into more socially acceptable behaviors. Who knows? That annoying

quirk may be the one thing that transfers into the world of work, leading to a productive and fulfilling career.

4. Enhance peer relationships.
We're all social beings and need continual interaction to develop. Depending on the stage of development, school offers children with ASD and their peers opportunities for building social networks and meaningful relationships. Having your child ride the bus or carpool with a classmate is a great start. Recess, which can be very difficult for children with ASD due to feelings of exclusion and loneliness, is an ideal time to have peers interact and support your child around shared interests. Remember, every relationship starts slowly, but even small interactions can be the beginning of a meaningful friendship.

5. Take advantage of resources.
A diagnosis of ASD, and its associated physical and mental health symptoms, can

take a toll on family functioning and harmony. Forming connections with other parents who are raising children with ASD is critical for optimizing your own sense of well-being. An occasional encouraging text from an ASD mom helped me to feel less alone during high stress points. There are exciting new developments in behavioral therapies and social support for ASD. Many nonprofits are partnering with ASD advocacy groups to provide weekend and week long camps for the entire family as well as respite for parents.

6. Prioritize self-care.
As parents, patience exits quickly when we're stressed and overwhelmed. Most ASD kids are sensitive to their parents' anxieties, which intensifies their own reactions. Keeping calm during meltdowns and practicing mindfulness help you to develop self-compassion during high stress periods, rather than feeling defeated. Simple activities such as meeting friends for lunch,

going to bed early, starting a new novel, or volunteering to take the kids out for some time so that your partner can have a break does wonders for pushing that reset button!

7. Accept your child for who they are.
The first step in acceptance is acknowledging the difficulties in parenting a child with ASD. Acceptance applies to both ourselves as parents and to our kids. Yes, parenting is very challenging, particularly during the early years. However, you need to work towards reducing judgment toward yourself or your child and, instead, cultivating compassion. Indeed, life would be much easier without autism in it, but this IS your life. Finding ways to help your child, and yourself, to adjust to your new normal will be beneficial.

Chapter 5: The Best Educational Toys for Autism in Toddlers

These are some of the Best Educational Toys for Toddlers with Autism to help them grow and develop in their own special way if your child has been diagnosed with autism.

Many parents are shocked, perplexed, and sometimes even relieved when their child is given an early diagnosis of autism.

One of the keys is being aware of the toddlers' early indicators of autism. Knowing what to do can also help you feel in control and assure you that you are doing everything in your power to support your kid while they deal with this difficulty.

The best thing you can do to help yourself process your own feelings about the diagnosis is sometimes just to know what kinds of toys to buy for toddlers who are autistic.

Sure, you probably already have toys on hand, but here are a few toddler educational toys that might be useful for a child who has just received an autism diagnosis.

Sure, you probably already have toys on hand, but here are a few toddler educational toys that can be useful for a child who has just received an autism diagnosis.

Educational Toys for Autism in Toddlers

Feel free to manufacture some of these toys if you can. Although some of them are not extremely complicated, some might not be DIY. However, if you need to buy toys or if your autistic child's grandparents are inquiring what to get him or her for Christmas or a birthday, point them to our list of the top educational toys for young autistic children.

Toddlers benefit greatly from toys that promote coordination and fine motor abilities. Toys that help toddlers with autism develop their fine motor abilities, however, can be even more advantageous. A toddler with autism frequently has delayed fine motor abilities. Therefore, having toys that promote fine motor abilities is quite advantageous.

And they don't have to be some fancy-dancy mess, just toys such as:

- Buttons
- Puzzles
- Latch and Hooks
- Cause and Effect (as the noise may also be rewarding)
- Play Dough or Slime

Imaginative play toys for toddlers on the spectrum can be things like:

- Mop & Broom Set
- Doctor Kit
- Kitchen Playset
- Camping Kit
- Farm Playset

You can also include a set of dress-up clothes and accessories. Just like a neurotypical toddler, autistic toddlers like to play dress-up and learn to understand their world through pretend play.

Interactive Toys for Toddlers with Autism

Interactive toys are some of the best educational and fun toys for a child. They usually stimulate and entertain the child so that they can learn while having fun. With an autistic toddler, they may also latch on to certain things with the toys. This is called stimming and yes, it is a typical behavior for people with autism.

In fact, I'll even bring up the dreaded fidget spinner.

Yes, I know, some parents are very much against them.

However, for a child on the spectrum, a fidget spinner can help with focusing. You, as a parent, should use your best judgment in this situation of course.

Other interactive toys an autistic toddler might like and benefit from include:

- Ball Poppers
- Gear Spinners
- Magnetic Drawing Boards
- Learning Piggy Bank
- Stacking Pegs
- Light-up Mushrooms
- Activity Cube

You can't really make these safely, because they have electrical components, unless, of course, you design and build electronic children's toys on the regular. But if you have grandparents asking what gifts they can get your autistic toddler, these are great for adding to that list.

Gross Motor Toys for Autistic Children

Other toys to consider for kids with autism include those that work more on the bigger muscle movements, too. Here's some of my favorite toys for autistic children:

- Pushing/Pulling or Filling/Emptying like:
- Wagons
- Trucks
- Carts
- Shopping Carts
- Buckets
- Balancers

Gross Motor Tools like what you'd find at an occupational therapist's office such as:

- Ball Pit
- Tricycles
- Balance Beams
- Trampoline
- Parachute
- Movement Scarves
- Scooter Boards
- Tunnel
- Hula Hoops
- Round Spot Markers
- Bean Bags
- Cones
- Saucer Swing

Other Toys Toddlers with Autism Might Like

It's wonderful that toddlers are inquisitive and enjoy touching and examining everything in their environment since this helps them build their hand-eye coordination. So feel free to choose toys that seem unique and are colorful to make things "interesting."

Children with autism will always choose action toys, cause and effect toys, and any activity that challenges their intellect. These toys end up being sensory toys to stimulate their sensory input.

Shape sorters, which are vibrant and engaging, may keep a kid occupied for hours and assist autistic children learn crucial abilities that aid in pattern recognition and problem-solving.

For the same reason—problem solving is really a superpower of many individuals affected by the autism spectrum disorder—stacking blocks, easy puzzles, and any toys that appear are also top on the list of entertaining and instructive toys for autistic children.

Colorful fridge magnets, books with noises and music, and other interactive toys are enjoyable for older young children. Any kind of imaginative play set, including dollhouses, airports, and garages, may be a fun and instructive method for your child to learn about the world and really aid in the development of social skills.

Buying Toys for Toddlers with Autism: A Word of Caution
Of course, keep in mind that your child will probably put items in their mouth. You'll still want toys with few little pieces that are age-appropriate.

To give you an example, when my daughter was younger, she had severe PICA. She needed to be continually observed since she was always mouthing things that weren't food. She still struggles with PICA, but not nearly as much as she did in the past.

Chapter 6: Top Tips to Prepare Your Autistic Toddler for Preschool

It is probable that you have used Early Intervention programs if you were given an early diagnosis of autism. My family's experience was the same, at least, although your circumstances could be different. However, if you're beginning to consider what will happen in preschool with your toddler who has autism, continue reading. You're about to start a journey of special needs advocacy.

My kid who has autism should attend preschool, right?
What happens when you obtain therapeutic services at home, if that is the case? There is nothing wrong with getting these treatments at a clinic or at home, for that matter. However, your youngster could require extra help.

For us, that meant calling a meeting of the Committee on Preschool Special Education in our community to discuss the next steps.

It was just a question of making adjustments to Sweet B's existing IFSP (Individual Family Service Plan) to better meet her evolving requirements.

In order to determine the amount of help she would require in her new setting, we were engaged in every stage of the process. But how would that affect Sweet B's transition? She had been at home with me up until this time while her therapists visited the household.

What program she would enroll in would come first. We may then develop a strategy for preparing our autistic kid for preschool after that.

Your preschool-aged autistic child

It's crucial to keep in mind that while your toddler may be autistic, they are still little children. When it comes to preparing a toddler for preschool, you may approach this in the same manner as you would for any other youngster.

Many parents sign their kids up for preschool programs without thinking about whether or not their kids are actually prepared for that level of education.

Children are entering preschool at earlier ages because many parents are anxious to give their child an advantage in the race to academic achievement. However, putting your child in preschool too early will hinder their education in the long run rather than providing them the head start you wanted.

What to Think About Before Enrolling Your Toddler with Autism in Preschool

How do you know whether your child is prepared for preschool? Examine the following three crucial areas: emotional growth, social development, and physical development.

You ought to examine the application itself as well. For instance, some programs are particularly designed for a young age group and focus more on play and social interaction than on formal teaching.

Some programs are designed to expose young children to schooling gradually and have relatively short time frames (just a few hours a week). However, in order to prepare kids for kindergarten, the typical preschool curriculum is often designed for kids between the ages of 3 and 4.

Even if your kid falls within the appropriate age range, it does not always indicate they are prepared for preschool.

A youngster may be set up for failure and a lifelong issue with school if they are forced into a formal school environment when they are not physically, socially, or emotionally prepared.

Physically, your kid should be able to take care of the majority of personal hygiene needs on their own or with help. This implies that the youngster must be capable of using the restroom and cleaning up after themselves (including unfastening and fastening clothing). Additionally, your youngster should be able to feed themself with little to no assistance.

Additionally, the kid should be able to concentrate on an activity for an extended period of time, such as drawing, as well as listen intently to a narrative or discussion for more than a few minutes.

Whether or if your child can keep the school schedule is another crucial aspect of physical development. Will your child's nutritional needs be met during the snack and lunch breaks? Will he be able to resist falling asleep or leaving until it is time to leave?

Children learn a lot about friendship and social connections in preschool, but if a child isn't ready for this degree of social engagement, it may be difficult on the child, class, and family.

Before entering preschool, children should have some prior experience playing with their classmates, learning to share and take turns, and resolving their conflicts. Taking instructions from people who are not their primary caretakers should also be practiced by kids.

For instance, a youngster who has only ever been in the care of a small number of relatives can find it difficult to adjust to being raised by an unfamiliar new adult.

When deciding if a kid is prepared for preschool, emotional development is yet another important factor to take into account. Is your kid prepared to leave behind home, parents, or a former daycare center? How does your kid handle unfamiliar surroundings and people?

You should delay enrolling your kid in preschool if you believe they are not ready in one or more of these crucial areas. It's possible that your youngster will have overcome those obstacles and be prepared to begin in a few months. Additionally, you may work with your child to improve the skills you believe need improvement, such as social skills or personal hygiene.

Many programs also allow you to progressively increase your child's engagement from a few hours per week to full participation.

Giving your child some time to adjust to a program is far preferable to pressing the problem because small children grow and develop at a phenomenal rate. Your kid won't notice the effects of those "lost" months on their schooling until later in life, but a pleasant preschool experience will have a long-lasting impact on learning and self-esteem.

The greatest approach to get your kid started on the path to academic achievement in preschool is to enroll them when they are ready, willing, and able.

You may also have a few toddler educational toys for autism on hand while you wait.

5 Tips to Help Prepare Your Autistic Toddler for Preschool

If at all possible, take a tour or multiple tours of your child's center and classroom. This will help them become familiar with the location. Introduce them to their teachers and support staff.

If your child thrives with visual aids, ask if it's okay to take pictures of the classroom and staff.

If your child's classroom will allow for it, ask if they would be okay with you creating a preschool schedule. Otherwise, work with your child's Speech Therapist to create one.

Starting preschool can be intimidating for any child but can be particularly difficult for autistic children. Helping them to become familiar with the new classroom and teachers could go a long way in reducing their anxiety.

Talk to classroom staff about what you do for meltdowns at home and ask what strategies that they use at school.

Message from the author

One of the key things to keep in mind here: your toddler is still a toddler. Your child is still a child. Just now, they happen to have an autism diagnosis.

Love them, unconditionally.

And hang in there moms & dads. Everything will work out fine.

9 798367 563108